FEATURED FALL PUMPKIN RECIPES

Gluten Free, Dairy Free, Soy Free and Nightshade Free

By Paula C. Henderson

Paula C. Henderson
Visit my website at

www.amazon.com/author/paulachenderson

Printed in the United States of America

First Printing: Aug 2020

ISBN- 9798693105928

Contents

ALL ABOUT PUMPKIN

The Backstory of the Pumpkin

Pumpkins are a part of the squash/gourd family. Native to North America, and Mexico. In some parts of the world pumpkins are called winter squash.

Squash is actually a fruit, but nutritionally more closely resembles a vegetable. Being harvested in October every year makes it the perfect 'fruit' for the holidays to come.

FEATURED FALL PUMPKIN RECIPES

Nutritional Value and Health Benefits

Pumpkins seeds

High in protein, zinc and copper as well as iron. Pumpkin seeds are also a good source of Vitamin E and a small bit of Vitamin K.

Pumpkin Flesh

Pumpkin is very healthy!

Very good source of Vitamin A. Just 12 carbs per one cup as compared to 27 carbs in one cup of sweet potatoes.

Besides being your best source of Vitamin A and beta-carotene, pumpkin is also a great source of Vitamin C, potassium, copper, all the B vitamins, iron and Vitamin E. It is also over 90% water which means it helps to keep you hydrated and all that water helps the body to absorb all the great vitamins and minerals the pumpkin has to offer.

Pumpkin is a great antioxidant. May help to boost your immune system, good for your eyes, skin and hair.

Having said all of that there are people who are allergic to pumpkin. So if you are serving pumpkin and someone says they are allergic please take it seriously and respect their desire to avoid the pumpkin.

How To Pick Out A Pumpkin For Cooking

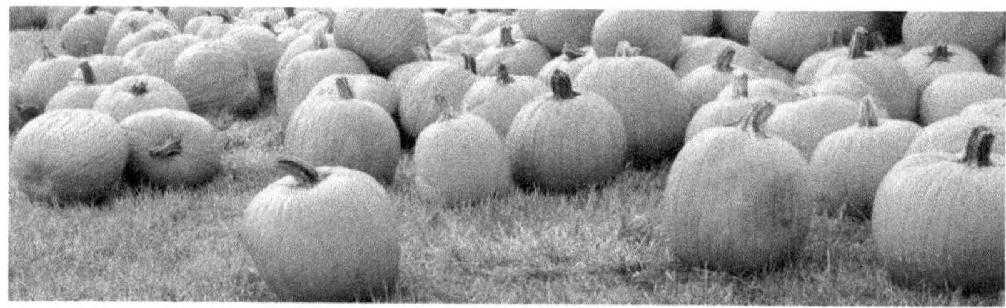

There are smaller 'sugar' pumpkins, as people like to call them that are generally found in the produce department and then there are jack-o-lanterns, or the larger pumpkins for carving that may be found outside or in a special display area. You can eat both kinds, but the smaller pumpkins are usually tastier.

Smaller pumpkins generally have a sweeter flesh. Wash well before cutting in half. Scrape out the seeds and unwanted guts of the pumpkin. Keeping the seeds to bake if you like those!

If you are going to use the pumpkin purely for puree I actually prefer to boil it until a knife slides easily through the rind. Allow to cool, cut in half, remove the seeds and guts. The rind will easily release from the flesh for you to then puree.

If you want to cube the cooked flesh I suggest the traditional baking method which will begin with cutting the raw pumpkin in half as mentioned earlier.

Place the raw pumpkin halves, rind side up, flesh side down, minus the seeds and bad guts, on a baking sheet. Pour a bit of water in the baking sheet.

Bake at 375 F for 45 minutes or until just turning tender. If you are going to puree the pumpkin, bake a full hour or so until very tender. Allow to cool and release the rind from the flesh.

To puree, simply place in your food processor and pulse until pureed. Add small amounts of water if needed.

Tip: if you will be using the pureed pumpkin for say, a pumpkin pie, it is highly recommended that you place the pureed pumpkin in a strainer and allow as much water to drain off as possible.

If you want to cube it, the pumpkin should be al dente or slightly underdone. It will finish cooking in whatever dish you will be using it in.

Pumpkin can be frozen but it is not recommended to take it through the canning process.

I read somewhere that in the Netherlands they dehydrate the rind (skin) and make pumpkin chips to eat. If you do not have a dehydrator use your oven:

Cut the cooked skin into chip size pieces. Sprinkle with salt and any seasoning you might like. Spread onto a baking sheet and bake at your ovens lowest temperate on bake with the oven door ajar for several hours. The number of hours will depend on your oven, and the region of the country you are in. Start them early morning in case you have to let them go throughout the day.

Pumpkin Seeds

Upon scooping out the seeds from a fresh pumpkin rinse them off, removing the strings, guts and any pulp. Spread the seeds out on a paper towel and allow them to completely dry.

An easy method to remove the guts from the seeds is to place it all in a large bowl of water or a sink of water. Massage the seeds under the water to easily dislodge all the unwanted excess.

Toss the cleaned, dried seeds with oil and salt and any other seasoning you find preferable.

Preheat the oven to 300 F degrees. Spread the seeds onto a baking sheet, being careful not to overcrowd them. Bake about 20 minutes or until they start to turn a golden brown. Stir the seeds around after ten minutes.

Seeds can be stored in an airtight container for about three days at room temperature.

BREAKFAST

PUMPKIN APPLE BREAKFAST PORRIDGE

- One can pumpkin puree
- One can coconut milk
- 2 medium apples, peeled and diced
- Dusting Spice mix*
- Honey to taste
- Dairy Free butter

Sauté apples in a saucepan in the DF butter. About five minutes. Add pumpkin puree and coconut milk along with the Dusting Spice Mix. Should be thick. Simmer about five to ten minutes or until the apples are tender.

Add honey to taste and top with DF butter and more of Spice Mix. Walnuts are also quite tasty atop your porridge.

PUMPKIN BREAD

- One 15 oz can pumpkin puree
- 1 and 1/3 cup Almond flour
- ¼ cup coconut flour
- ¼ cup flaxseed meal
- 1 tablespoon xanthum gum
- 1 tablespoon cornstarch or arrowroot
- 1 tablespoon pumpkin pie spice
- 1 tablespoon baking powder
- ½ teaspoon salt
- 6 tablespoons Dairy Free butter or solid coconut oil
- 1 cup sugar
- 2 teaspoons apple cider vinegar
- 4 eggs

For best results start by regrinding your flaxseed meal or you can put it in your blender and pulse it a few times before beginning the recipe.

Combine the almond flour, coconut flour, flaxseed meal, xantham gum, cornstarch, pumpkin pie spice, baking powder and salt. Set aside.

Cream the butter or coconut oil with sugar until fluffy. Add vinegar and add the eggs one at a time. The batter will appear to break.

Add the flour mixture to the eggs and butter about one half cup at a time. Alternating adding spoonfuls of the pumpkin puree. Until you have combined all of the flour and pumpkin puree into the creamed butter, eggs and sugar.

Pour the batter into a greased loaf pan. Be sure it is distributed evenly.

Bake in a Pre-Heated 350 F oven for about 60 minutes. Should be golden brown and a toothpick should come out clean. Cover with foil while baking if it starts turning too brown before cooking time is up.

It is absolutely necessary to allow this bread to cool in the loaf pan for at least 20 minutes before trying to remove or even cut. Do not glaze until after it has cooled.

Glaze

- 1 teaspoon ginger
- 1 tablespoon water
- 6 tablespoons powdered sugar
- Pinch of salt

Mix the ginger, water, powdered sugar and salt together.

Add more water if needed for a drizzling icing consistency.

If it is too thin add more powdered sugar.

PUMPKIN PANCAKES

- 1 cup brown rice flour
- ½ cup tapioca starch
- 2 tablespoons baking powder
- ¼ teaspoon xanthan gum
- ¼ teaspoon salt
- ½ can pumpkin puree (about 8 ounces)
- 1 teaspoon vanilla
- 2 tablespoons maple syrup or honey
- ¼ cup dairy free milk
- 1 large egg, 1 egg yolk

Mix all ingredients together. If the batter seems too thick add more milk.

CONDIMENTS

13

HONEY MUSTARD PUMPKIN DRESSING

- ½ cup pumpkin puree
- ½ cup apple cider vinegar
- ½ cup canola or olive oil
- 6 tablespoons honey
- 3 tablespoons Dijon mustard
- One garlic clove, smashed and minced
- ½ teaspoon salt
- ½ teaspoon black pepper
- ½ teaspoon thyme

Put all of the ingredients, except the oil, in the blender and pulse a few times to blend well.

Add the oil in a slow stream while running the blender to combine well.

Store in the refrigerator in a glass jar for up to one week.

Shake well before serving.

PUMPKIN DIP

This gets great reviews!

- 12 ounces dairy free cream cheese (I like Kite Hill brand)
- ¾ cup pumpkin puree
- 2 tablespoons cumin
- 1/8 teaspoon garlic powder
- 1 teaspoon coriander
- 1/3 cup dried beef (Hormel Dried Beef found in a jar)
- 1/8 cup minced scallions or green onions
- ½ cup sliced green olives (pimento removed if you are avoiding nightshades)

Work with softened cream cheese.

Cream together the cream cheese, pumpkin puree, cumin, coriander, and garlic powder.

Chop the dried beef into bite size pieces and add to the cream cheese mixture along with the olives and scallions.

Cover and chill at least an hour before serving.

Serve with raw vegetables, corn and tortilla chips.

PUMPKIN JAM

- 1 cup frozen cranberries
- 1/3 cup pumpkin puree
- 3 tablespoons honey
- ½ tablespoon cinnamon

Heat cranberries in a saucepan until thawed and somewhat saucy. Simmer about ten minutes and stir often.

Add the pumpkin puree, honey and cinnamon. Combine well and allow to simmer about five to ten minutes. Remove from heat and allow to cool.

This makes a wonderful jam for toast and muffins, or a topping for pancakes and waffles.

PUMPKIN PIE SPICE

I just wanted to include this since it is used in so many of the recipes and in case you cannot find the blend in the store:

- 4 teaspoons cinnamon
- 1 teaspoon ground cloves
- 2 teaspoons ginger
- ½ teaspoon nutmeg

DESSERTS

NO-BAKE PUMPKIN CHEESECAKE

Gluten Free Graham Cracker Crust (Mid-del brand makes one available in most stores)

- One 15 ounce can coconut milk, chilled and shaken
- 16 ounces DF cream cheese
- One 15 oz can pumpkin puree
- 1 cup powdered sugar
- 1 teaspoon vanilla
- 1 teaspoon cinnamon
- ½ teaspoon nutmeg
- ¼ teaspoon salt

Beat the coconut milk until thickened. Set aside. You will fold this in shortly.

In a glass bowl beat the softened cream cheese until light and fluffy.

Add the pumpkin and beat until smooth and well combined. Add the powdered sugar and beat again until combined.

Add the vanilla, cinnamon, nutmeg and salt.

Fold in the whipped coconut milk.

Transfer filling into the GF crust. Refrigerate at least 4 hours. Serve with DF whipped cream topping.

PECAN PUMPKIN PIE

Have your favorite prebaked gluten free pie crust on hand.

- One 15 ounce can pumpkin puree
- 2 medium eggs, beaten
- 3.5 ounces coconut milk fat (canned coconut milk; chilled and drained)
- 1 teaspoon pumpkin pie spice
- ¼ teaspoon nutmeg
- 6 ounces brown sugar
- 2 ounces honey
- 4 ounces chopped pecans

Beat together pumpkin puree, eggs, coconut fat, spices and the sugar.

Pour into pie crust. Bake in a 375 F. preheated oven about 45 minutes or until set.

To make the sticky pecan topping:

Spray a saucepan with non-stick cooking spray.

Put the sugar and honey in the saucepan and heat over low/med heat until sugars are dissolved. Turn the heat up just enough to bring to a simmer; add pecans and stir to coat well.
Pour over the pie. Allow to cool.

PUMPKIN BARS

Filling:

- 29 ounce can pumpkin puree
- 1 and ¼ cups almond or coconut milk (carton, not can)
- 4 large eggs
- ½ cup maple syrup
- ½ cup coconut sugar (or white granulated sugar)
- 1 teaspoon cinnamon
- 1 teaspoon nutmeg
- 1 teaspoon salt
- ½ teaspoon cloves

Crust:

- 1/3 cup rice flour
- 1/3 cup sorghum flour
- 1/3 cup tapioca flour (starch)
- ½ cup quick cook oats
- 1 teaspoon xanthan gum
- ½ cup shortening (coconut works well here)
- ½ cup sugar (coconut or white)

Topping: chopped pecans (optional)

Preheat oven to 350 F

Line a 9x13 baking dish with parchment paper.

To make the crust:

Combine rice flour, sorghum flour, tapioca starch, oats, sugar and the xanthan gum. Cut in the shortening. Should resemble coarse crumbs.

Press into the prepared baking pan over the parchment paper. Bake in a preheated 350 F for 20 minutes.

While that is baking make the filling:

In a large mixing bowl combine the pumpkin puree, milk, eggs, syrup, sugar, cinnamon, nutmeg, salt, and the cloves. Using a mixer, beat until smooth.

Pour into crust.

Return to the 350 oven and bake 45 minutes.

PUMPKIN CAKE

- 2 cups all-purpose gluten free flour blend (There are many on the market but it is challenging to find one without potato starch which is a nightshade. You will find an All-Purpose Gluten Free Flour blend you can make at home below to mix up and store just like you would any other flour)
- 2 teaspoons baking powder
- 1 teaspoon baking soda
- ½ teaspoon salt
- 1.5 teaspoon cinnamon
- 2 teaspoons Pumpkin Pie Spice
- 1 cup granulated sugar

- 1 cup canola oil
- 4 large eggs
- One 15 oz can pumpkin puree

Cream Cheese Frosting:

- 4 ounces DF cream cheese softened
- ½ cup DF butter
- 3.5 cups powdered sugar
- 1 teaspoon vanilla
- 2-4 tablespoons water or DF milk

Preheat oven to 350 F

Combine the dry ingredients in a glass bowl.

Add pumpkin, eggs, and vanilla to the dry ingredients. Mix well.

Pour into a greased 9x13 baking pan.

Bake in preheated oven 35-40 minutes. Check for doneness by inserting a toothpick.

Allow to cool completely before icing.

To make the icing: Using a mixer, beat all of the Cream Cheese Frosting ingredients together.

All-Purpose Gluten Free Flour:

- 2 cups white rice flour
- 2 cups brown rice flour
- 1 cup arrowroot starch (or cornstarch)
- ½ cup tapioca starch

PUMPKIN CUPCAKES

- One 15 oz can pumpkin puree
- ½ cup white granulated sugar
- ¼ cup light brown sugar
- 2 large eggs
- 1 egg yolk
- 1 teaspoon vanilla
- 1 can coconut milk (shaken)
- ¾ cup gluten free all-purpose flour blend
- 2 teaspoons pumpkin pie spice
- ½ teaspoon pumpkin pie spice
- ½ teaspoon salt
- ¼ teaspoon baking soda
- ¼ teaspoon baking powder

- Dairy Free coconut milk whipped cream

Preheat oven to 350 F. Line muffin tins with paper liners and spray generously with non stick spray.

In a large bowl combine: pumpkin, sugar, brown sugar, eggs, yolk, vanilla, and the coconut milk.

In a separate bowl sift together the flour blend, spices, salt, baking soda and the baking powder. Transfer to the wet ingredients and combine well whisking quickly leaving some air bubbles. Set aside.

Fill the muffin tin cups almost to the top. Bake in preheated oven approximately 25 minutes.
It is very important to allow the cupcakes to not only cool, but to then, after they have cooled to refrigerate them for one full hour.
Top with your favorite icing or dairy free whipped topping.

PUMPKIN MOUSSE

- One 3.4 ounce box INSTANT vanilla pudding (the instant pudding is GF, DF, SF & Nightshade Free but the prepared pudding cups are not)
- One 15 oz can pumpkin puree
- ½ teaspoon cinnamon
- 1 teaspoon pumpkin pie spice
- ½ teaspoon salt
- 2 tablespoons maple syrup or honey
- ½ teaspoon vanilla
- 1 cup coconut milk (from the refrigerated carton)
- 1.5 cups canned coconut milk fat (canned coconut milk that has been chilled and drained leaving you with the fat only)

Whisk together in a glass bowl, pudding mix, spices and salt.

Add the pumpkin, syrup, vanilla and refrigerated coconut milk. Set aside.

In a separate glass bowl, whip the canned coconut fat into peaks. Fold 2/3 of this into the other bowl with the pudding mix and pumpkin.

Spoon into serving dishes and top with the remaining whipped coconut fat.

PUMPKIN PIE

- Gluten free crust
- One 15 oz can pumpkin puree
- 2 large eggs, beaten
- 1 cup coconut milk (carton or shaken can)
- ½ cup maple syrup
- 1 teaspoon cinnamon
- ½ teaspoon ginger
- 1/8 teaspoon cloves
- 1/8 teaspoon salt

Preheat oven to 425 F

Mix the pumpkin, eggs, milk, maple syrup, cinnamon, ginger, cloves, and the salt.

Pour into the crust and sprinkle the top lightly with white granulated sugar.

Bake ten minutes. Then, turn the oven down to 350 F. and continue to bake for another 35 minutes.

Remove when a skin forms on top of the pumpkin ad the crust is just lightly golden brown.

Your best bet is a crust that has not been pre-baked. Allow the pie to cool before refrigerating to chill. If you use a pre-baked GF pie crust, follow the directions on the packaging.

PUMPKIN RUM TART

Filling:

- 1 ¼ cup pumpkin puree
- 2 tablespoons dark rum
- ¾ cup sugar (coconut sugar works nicely)
- 1 teaspoon vanilla
- 2 large eggs
- 1 teaspoon cinnamon
- ¼ cup maple syrup
- 1 cup coconut milk (refrigerated carton or canned that has been shaken well)

To make the crust:

- 1 cup Almond flour
- 1 cup GF graham cracker crumbs
- 1/3 cup unsweetened cocoa powder
- ½ cup coconut sugar
- 1/3 cup melted coconut oil or melted DF butter

Preheat oven to 350 F. Grease tart pan.

In a large bowl mix all of the ingredients for the filling. Set aside.

Make the crust: combine the flour, crumbs, cocoa, and sugar. Add coconut oil or butter. Mix well.

Press into the tart pan. Pour the filling into the crust. Bake in preheated oven for 25 minutes. Allow to cool completely. Move to the refrigerator and chill.

Serve chilled.

DRINKS

BANANA PUMPKIN SMOOTHIE

- One cup pumpkin puree
- One medium ripe banana, frozen
- One cup dairy free milk. I like coconut milk (the carton, not the canned) but almond milk would absolutely be okay too.
- 1 tablespoon chia seeds
- ½ teaspoon vanilla
- ½ teaspoon pumpkin pie spice
- 2-3 tablespoon maple syrup or honey
- 4-6 ice cubes or freeze some DF milk the night before, and use that instead of water ice cubes. (Yes, on top of the frozen cubes of milk you would still use the one cup of dairy free milk mentioned above)

Place all of the ingredients in the blender. Pulse until smooth and creamy. Enjoy!

CHOCOLATE PUMPKIN SHAKE

- ½ cups pumpkin puree
- One 15 oz can coconut milk (the entire can, shaken) - chilled
- 1-2 tablespoons carob powder or unsweetened cocoa powder
- 1-4 tablespoon honey
- 1 teaspoon cinnamon
- ½ teaspoon ginger
- ½ teaspoon vanilla extract or vanilla flavoring

Chill the entire can of coconut milk the night before.

Combine all of your ingredients into the blender. Add refrigerated, carton coconut milk if you need to thin it out. Sweetener is to taste.

DUSTING SPICE MIX

- 4 teaspoons cinnamon
- 1 teaspoon cloves
- ½ teaspoon nutmeg
- 1-2 teaspoons white or brown sugar

Combine well for dusting atop cocoa, tea, coffee, latte's and smoothies.

PUMPKIN APPLE CIDER

- 4 cups apple cider
- 1 cup pumpkin puree

Bring the apple cider and pumpkin puree to a low simmer over medium heat.

Simmer about ten minutes. I like to use a whisk for best results.

I have had some reviews that say they like to actually simmer with a lemon slice.

Dust with Dusting Spice Mix or a squeeze of lemon juice to brighten it up before serving.

PUMPKIN SMOOTHIE

- 12 oz coffee
- 8 oz coconut milk, refrigerated carton or canned.
- ¼ cup pumpkin puree
- 2-3 Tbs maple syrup
- 1 tsp cinnamon
- ½ tsp ginger
- ¼ tsp cloves

Brew your coffee the night before, let cool and pour into ice cube trays to freeze.

Add frozen coffee cubes, coconut milk, pumpkin, maple syrup and spices to blender.

Blend until smooth.
Pour into a glass, top with cinnamon and serve.

PUMPKIN SPICED LATTE

- 1 cup Coconut Milk (refrigerated in the carton, not canned)
- 2 tablespoons pumpkin puree
- 1 tablespoon maple syrup or honey
- ½ teaspoon Pumpkin Pie Spice
- 1 teaspoon vanilla
- ¼ cup hot espresso or hot coffee
- Dairy Free Whipped Cream for topping

Over medium heat, in a saucepan, heat the milk, pumpkin, syrup, spice and the vanilla. Whisking to mix well.

Remove from heat and use an immersion blender to make your drink frothy!

Pour your fresh, hot espresso or black coffee into a mug and then add your pumpkin milk mixture from the saucepan.
Whether you stir or not at this point is up to you. Many do not.

Top with DF whipped topping!

PUMPKIN TEA (HOT)

- 8 ounce brewed black or orange pekoe tea
- 2 ounces coconut milk (carton or canned)
- 4 tablespoons pureed pumpkin
- 1 teaspoon maple syrup or honey
- ½ teaspoon cinnamon
- 1/8 teaspoon cloves
- 1/8 teaspoon vanilla

Combine all ingredients in a blender. Blend until very smooth! Should be somewhat frothy. Reheat if you need to and enjoy by adding a bit of Dusting Spice Mix.

Dusting Spice Mix:

- 4 teaspoons cinnamon
- 1 teaspoon cloves
- ½ teaspoon nutmeg
- 1-2 teaspoons white or brown sugar

Combine well for dusting atop cocoa, tea, coffee, latte's and smoothies.

TURMERIC PUMPKIN SIPPER

If you are looking for an opportunity to add turmeric into your diet give this a try. It's a nice change from hot cocoa on a cold morning or afternoon.

- 1.5 cups coconut milk (refrigerated carton)
- 2 tablespoons pumpkin puree
- 2 teaspoons turmeric
- 1 teaspoon Dusting Spice Mix (see recipe above)

Combine all ingredients (including the Dusting Spice Mix) in a saucepan. Heat through. Strain and serve hot.

Honey to taste for sweetener

ENTREES AND SIDES

CAULIFLOWER PUMPKIN CASSEROLE

- 2 cups Cream of Pumpkin Soup (recipe in this book under entrees)
- 1 head cauliflower
- One 8 ounce container dairy free cream cheese or dairy free shredded cheese you like! (I like the tartness of the cream cheese. It reminds me of feta.)
- ½ cup gluten free bread crumbs

Preheat oven to 400 degrees F.

Cut cauliflower into bite size pieces and boil until tender. Drain.

Make the Cream of Pumpkin Soup.

Combine the soup and the cooked cauliflower. Taste and adjust salt and pepper.

Transfer to a baking dish.

Dollop the top with cream cheese or top with your favorite dairy free shredded cheese.

Then top with gluten free bread crumbs.

Bake in preheated oven about 20 minutes or until cheese is melted.

Hit it with the broiler if you need to but stand by so as not to burn.

Presumably you are placing this in the oven while the cauliflower and the soup is already heated.

If not, because you made those items the day before, I usually combine the two and heat in a saucepan first or you could microwave them before building the casserole and baking.

CAULIFLOWER AND PUMPKIN MASH

- One head raw cauliflower
- 3 cups chicken broth
- One 15 oz can pumpkin puree
- 4 ounces DF cream cheese (I use Kite Hill brand)
- ½ teaspoon garlic powder
- 1/8 teaspoon thyme
- 1 teaspoon salt
- ½ teaspoon black pepper

Boil the cauliflower in the chicken broth until very tender. Drain.

Add the pumpkin, room temperature cream cheese, garlic, thyme, salt and pepper to the drained cauliflower.

Using a mixer, mix until whipped like potatoes.

If too thick add just a small amount of plain water.

CREAM OF PUMPKIN SOUP

- One 15 oz can pumpkin puree
- 1 small onion
- 1 garlic clove, smashed and minced
- 5 white button mushrooms, sliced or diced
- 2 teaspoons salt
- 1 teaspoon thyme
- 2 cups chicken broth
- 1 tablespoon apple cider vinegar
- Black pepper to taste

Sauté the onion and garlic in oil or dairy free butter in a saucepan.

Add mushrooms, and salt. Stir around to coat well and cook just a few minutes until the mushrooms start to soften.

Add the pumpkin puree and the chicken broth. Combing well.

Add salt, pepper, thyme and vinegar. Some people find adding a pinch of nutmeg really adds something to the dish if you would like to give that a try.

Allow to simmer, covered, about 15 minutes or so until the onions and mushrooms are softened through. Serve hot.

This not only makes a lovely soup but makes a great sauce on gluten free pasta or spaghetti squash.

EASY PUMPKIN SOUP IN A HURRY

- One 15 ounce can pumpkin puree
- One cup chicken broth
- 1 teaspoon salt
- 1 teaspoon cumin
- ½ teaspoon black pepper
- 1 tablespoon apple cider vinegar

Using a whisk, combine all ingredients in a saucepan and heat through.

Perfect on a cold weeknight when you've had a long day but also elegant enough to serve to company as part of a full course dinner.

LENTIL PUMPKIN SOUP (SLOW COOKER)

- 2 cups bite size cubed pumpkin
- 1 cup dried lentils
- 1 medium onion, diced in food chopper
- 2 celery stalks, diced in food chopper
- 3 garlic cloves, smashed and minced
- 1 tablespoons cumin
- 1 teaspoon coriander
- 1 teaspoon garlic powder
- 1 teaspoon salt
- ½ teaspoon black pepper
- ½ teaspoon thyme
- ½ teaspoon ginger
- 1/8 teaspoon nutmeg
- 4 cups chicken stock
- 2 tablespoons apple cider vinegar

Place all ingredients in the slow cooker. Cook on low 6-8 hours. Have more chicken broth on hand in case you need it half or three quarters way through cooking.

PUMPKIN CHILI

- 1 pound ground beef
- 2 celery stalks, diced in chopper with onion
- 1 onion, diced
- 1 tablespoon GF worcestershire
- 2 tablespoons cumin
- 1 tablespoons coriander
- 1 teaspoon garlic powder
- 1 teaspoon onion powder
- 1 teaspoon salt
- ½ teaspoon black pepper
- ½ teaspoon lemon pepper
- 1/8 teaspoon nutmeg
- One 15 oz can pumpkin puree
- One 15 oz can pinto or black beans
- 1 cup carrot puree:

Carrot Puree:

- One 15 ounce can carrots with liquid or replace liquid with half cup water if you prefer
- 1 teaspoon beef bouillon
- 2 tablespoons apple cider vinegar
- ½ teaspoon salt

Combine all four ingredients in the blender and blend until quite smooth. Should smell like tomato sauce.

Brown the ground beef, onion and celery, in a large skillet or large saucepan you will use for the chili. Half way through browning add cumin, coriander, garlic powder, onion powder, nutmeg, salt and pepper. Add pumpkin, carrot puree, beans to the ground beef mixture.

Cover and allow to simmer at least 30 minutes. If you like your chili more soupy add one cup chicken broth or one cup water and one teaspoon chicken bouillon.

PUMPKIN CORNBREAD

- 2 cups GF cornmeal
- 1 teaspoon baking soda
- 1 teaspoon salt
- 1 teaspoon cinnamon
- ½ teaspoon pumpkin spice
- 1 large egg, beaten
- ¼ cup melted coconut oil or DF butter
- One can pumpkin puree
- ½ cup DF plain yogurt (not vanilla!)

Preheat oven to 350 F and grease a 9 inch square pan

Mix together the cornmeal, sugar, salt, baking soda, cinnamon, pumpkin spice.

Add in the egg, pumpkin puree and plain yogurt.

Stream in the melted coconut oil or you could use melted DF butter; stirring the entire time.

Bake 20 minutes or until the top turns a golden brown and center is set.

Allow to cool, in the pan.

PUMPKIN PEAR SOUP

- One 15 ounce can pumpkin puree
- 1 cup chicken broth
- 1 medium/large pear, peeled and chopped
- 1/8 cup diced onion
- 2 garlic cloves, smashed and minced
- 2 tablespoons DF butter
- ½ teaspoon ginger
- ¼ teaspoon cinnamon
- ½ teaspoon salt

Melt the butter in a saucepan. Add onion and cook until softened. About five minutes.

Add the garlic. Stir around and cook two full minutes.

Add the broth, pumpkin, pears, cinnamon, ginger and salt. Bring this to a low boil.

Cover and simmer on low for 40 minutes.

Remove from heat when the pears are tender and mushy. Allow to cool. Transfer to blender and pulse until smooth and creamy.

This soup is wonderful at room temperature. If you feel it needs sweetened, add a bit of honey before serving.

The sweetness will vary depending on the sweetness of the pumpkin and pear used each time prepared.

PUMPKIN SLOPPY JOE

- 1 pound ground beef
- One 15 ounce can pumpkin puree
- 1 medium onion, minced (I like to use my food chopper)
- 2 celery stalks, minced with onion
- 1 teaspoon salt
- ½ teaspoon black pepper
- 1 tablespoon beef bouillon
- 1 tablespoon GF Worcestershire
- 1/8 teaspoon liquid smoke
- 2 tablespoons apple cider vinegar
- 1 tablespoon sugar
- 1 teaspoon garlic powder
- ½ teaspoon onion powder
- ¼ teaspoon celery seed

- Gluten Free Hamburger Buns

Brown the ground beef, onion and celery.

Add the pumpkin puree, salt, pepper, beef bouillon, Worcestershire, vinegar, liquid smoke, sugar, garlic, onion powder and the celery seed to the ground beef mixture in the skillet.

Continue to cook. Simmer about 15 minutes. Taste and adjust salt, vinegar and sugar if needed.

Serve hot on buns.

PUMPKIN WEDGES

Peel and trim a fresh pumpkin. If you find this difficult, you can make the job a bit easier by boiling the whole pumpkin until a paring knife can begin to penetrate the skin.

This will not cook the pumpkin flesh completely (unless you leave it boil), but it will help to make cutting the whole pumpkin in half or peeling off the skin to cut wedges and then finish roasting the flesh in the oven. So as soon as your paring knife can penetrate drain off the hot water. Allow to cool enough to handle the pumpkin.

Back to the recipe: Peel and trim the pumpkin into large wedges. Similar to how you might cut wedges of an acorn squash.

Toss the wedges in oil, salt, cumin and lemon pepper. Spread onto a baking sheet making sure not to crowd. Use two baking sheets if you need to.

Bake in a preheated 400 F oven for half hour; turning halfway through baking.

You can absolutely swap out the seasoning here for cinnamon or go savory with thyme and sage.

ROASTED PUMPKIN AND BRUSSELS SPROUTS WITH SAUSAGE

- 1 pound breakfast sausage (I like Farmland Original Breakfast Sausage which is GF and nightshade free.
- 2 cups cubed bite size raw pumpkin
- 1 cup raw, halved brussels sprouts
- ½ cup olive oil
- 4 garlic cloves, smashed and minced
- 2 tablespoons apple cider vinegar
- 1 teaspoon salt
- ½ teaspoon black pepper

In a bowl combine the oil, garlic, vinegar, salt and pepper. Toss the pumpkin and brussels sprouts in the oil mixture. Spread out onto a baking sheet. Use two or three baking sheets if you need to in order to spread out your vegetables and avoiding crowding.

Bake the vegetables in a preheated 400 F oven until tender through and slightly golden brown.

While the vegetables are roasting in the oven brown the sausage into crumbles, like you would ground beef. You could use ground pork if you prefer. Season with salt, pepper, sage, cumin, and coriander.

Combine the cooked vegetables with the sausage in the skillet. A fresh squeeze of lemon juice before serving will brighten the dish.

SAUSAGE AND PUMPKIN SAGE STUFFING

- 1.5 cups fresh cooked pumpkin, smashed (great opportunity if you have some in the freezer)
- 2 tablespoons DF butter
- 1 pound ground pork
- 1 cup fresh chopped fennel
- 1 leek, chopped
- 1 small white onion, chopped
- 1 tablespoons sage
- 1 teaspoon marjoram
- ¼ teaspoon salt

Brown the ground pork. Halfway through add the onion, leek, and fennel to sauté with the pork.

Add the remaining ingredients once the sausage has cooked through and vegetables have softened.

Taste and adjust salt and sage. I will sometimes add a bit of garlic powder.

Transfer to a greased casserole dish.

Bake in a 350 F oven for 20 minutes.

SLOW COOKER APRICOT CHICKEN WITH PUMPKIN

- 3 cups cubed pumpkin (raw)
- 3 tablespoons cooking oil
- 4 boneless, skinless chicken breasts, cut into bite size pieces
- 1 small onion, chopped into bite size pieces
- 2 garlic cloves, smashed and minced
- ½ cup dried apricots
- ¼ cup chicken broth
- ½ cup apricot preserves
- 1 tablespoons lemon juice
- 1 teaspoon ginger
- ½ teaspoon cinnamon
- 1 teaspoon salt
- 1 teaspoon black pepper

Place all of the ingredients in the slow cooker. Cover and cook on low at least 5 hours or until the chicken is cooked through.

If you find you have a lot of broth and would prefer it thickened, just remove a small about of the broth and whisk with some corn starch or arrowroot to make a roux.

Bring the crock pot to a boil and return the roux while whisking.

SPAGHETTI SQUASH WITH PUMPKIN SAGE SAUCE

You could, of course, substitute your favorite Gluten Free pasta instead of using the spaghetti squash.

Prepare your pasta or spaghetti squash as you normally would. While that is cooking prepare the sauce:

- 14 fresh sage leaves
- 2 tablespoons cooking oil

- 1 small to med Onion, diced
- 2 Garlic cloves, smashed and minced
- 1 tablespoon Cornstarch or arrowroot
- 3 slices Bacon, cooked crispy
- One 15 oz can pumpkin puree
- ¾ cup chicken broth
- Juice of half a lemon
- ½ teaspoon nutmeg

'Fry' the sage leaves in the oil briefly. Only about 2-3 minutes.

Be careful to not let it burn or even get too browned or it could turn bitter.

Gently stir the sage leaves in the simmering oil, remove from skillet and set aside.

Using the same skillet: sauté the onion and garlic until softened. Sprinkle with cornstarch and stir around to coat. Set aside. While in a separate skillet or oven, cook your crispy bacon.

Combine chicken broth, pumpkin puree, lemon and nutmeg in a saucepan.

Bring to a low boil. Allow to simmer, uncovered, about ten minutes.

Add the fried sage. Stir around to combine.

Transfer to the skillet with the onion and garlic.

Whisk to combine well and heat through. Should thicken somewhat.

Add crispy, crumbled bacon last, just before serving.

THAI PUMPKIN SOUP

- One 15 ounce can pumpkin puree
- ½ cup chicken broth
- ½ cup coconut milk
- 1 tablespoons minced onion
- 1 teaspoon ginger
- 1 tablespoon minced lemongrass
- 1 teaspoon salt
- 1 teaspoon cumin
- ½ teaspoon black pepper

- Some fresh chopped cilantro

Using a whisk, combine all ingredients, except cilantro, in a saucepan and heat through while whisking. Garnish with cilantro and a squeeze of lime juice.

Check out all published works by Paula C. Henderson on her Amazon author's page:

amazon.com/author/paulachenderson